MW00946696

# Nutrition Facts for Kids

## Teaching Children the Facts about Nutrition

by

Maryse A. Rouffaer

Copyright © 2013 Maryse A. Rouffaer
All rights reserved.

ISBN: 1493511815

ISBN 13: 9781493511815

Library of Congress Control Number: 2013919316
CreateSpace Independent Publishing Platform
North Charleston, South Carolina

NutritionFactsForKids® owns the copyright to the contents of this book. Readers are permitted to copy parts of the content, provided the original source is cited and/or an executable hyperlink to the source www.nutritionfactsforkids.com is given. It is prohibited to sell this book to third parties.

To all kids who want to learn about nutrition and
to
Philippe and Victor

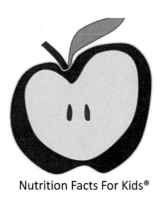

Nutrition Facts For Kids®

Written by Maryse Rouffaer

Edited by Virginia E. Ward

Illustrated by Maryse Rouffaer

# Contents

# Why? 🍎

Why is it important to write a book on what and how to eat? It's surprising, but many people are not sure which foods are best for us, and why.

## MULTIGRAIN IS ALWAYS HEALTHY, RIGHT?

## FAT-FREE MARGARINE MUST BE BETTER THAN FATTY BUTTER, RIGHT?

## ADDED VITAMINS AND ADDED FIBER SOUNDS REALLY GREAT, TRUE?

No! No! No!

With plenty of food everywhere and grocery stores that give you more choices than ever before, you would think that it would be easier than ever to prepare a healthy diet?

NOT THE CASE!

It is important for children to know how they can ensure their own good health and how to better understand the factors that influence it. A common saying about nutrition is, 'you are what you eat'. For children, this means they grow their bodies and brains with the food they consume! It is important to grow using good, nutritious food to ensure excellent health.

Most children do not decide what groceries to buy and probably don't cook the family meals, but most parents want their children to be educated consumers to prepare them for adulthood. Just as a parent chooses the best doctor and the best school for their children, parents also want their children to be educated about the best choices for good nutrition. This book explains why people are confused about what and how to eat. It will help you understand the challenges to eating well and will empower you to improve your nutrition choices and take control of your health.

With so much information and so many choices to make when we go food shopping, it's important to know which foods to choose. That's why this book is such a great idea!

# 1   Not too long ago...

Imagine you lived about 100 years ago. The world was a very different place and looked very different too. There were no busy airports or highways, no huge shopping centers or supermarkets, no television, no computers...

Life today is much more convenient. You can quickly travel from your country to another by car or plane, and machines now do a lot of work for us. Sewing machines, washers and dryers, dishwashers and vacuum cleaners are all forms of progress most people like. If you have to find your way, you can use a Global Positioning System (GPS). If your school is far away, you don't have to walk, but you can arrive by car in minutes! If you need an answer to a difficult question you just use your computer to find the answer in seconds!

People lived very differently not too long ago. Imagine someone from that time being in a big supermarket today. What foods would they recognize?

People who lived 100 years ago would only recognize some of the fruits and vegetables, the meat, fish and bread, but they would not understand the miracle of strawberries in December. In the dairy section they would recognize the whole milk, yogurt and cheese, but the pink or brown milk would be a mystery. They would not recognize boxed cereals as real foods and they would not have a clue what some of our snack foods are, based on the ingredients listed on the packages. They would not understand the phrase 'made with real fruit'; what 'unreal' fruit could there be? They would also not understand why people buy water and why it is so expensive! In their time, water was not as polluted as it is today and it was safe to drink it from a tap or a river.

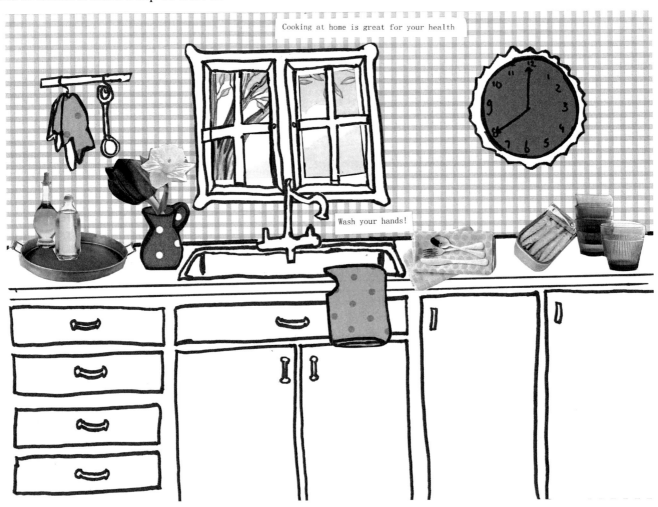

People from that time ate meat and dairy from the chickens, cows, sheep and goats that lived on their land. They grew their own vegetables, herbs and fruit and would go to near-by markets to buy whatever they didn't grow themselves. They knew where their food came from and only ate food that was in season. In general, they ate less and ate small portions of meat only as a treat. They cooked their own meals and took time to eat with their families at their dinner tables and not in front of a television or hurried in a fast food drive- thru!

Today, most of us do not grow our own food. We buy it in supermarkets where it has been purchased from all over the world. We do not know the people who grew our food, nor do we know the distance our food traveled from the farm to our table. We are not concerned about the availability of strawberries in December because they come from farms in warm places far away. We talk about comfort foods, convenience foods, microwaveable and freezable foods. We have no idea where these foods were grown, who prepared them or what ingredients went into their creation. Sometimes we do not even know if the food came from a plant, an animal, out of a laboratory, or a combination of all three!

Unfortunately all these new food choices have not resulted in healthier people. Today, people eat too much food, but they still do not get enough nutrients. They become undernourished and experience more chronic diseases, such as heart disease and diabetes, at an earlier age. All these new food choices have resulted in confusion about what to eat and how to cook. We no longer have the life skills of the people who lived 100 years ago, and contradictory to what you might think, with the abundance of food available today, it is really hard to find nutritious, real food.

Let's review:

1. A century and longer ago, people typically ate less and what they ate was local, fresh and in season! Today's food is not necessarily fresh or local or in season.

2. People nowadays eat more and their food is different.

3. Nowadays, people have many food choices from all over the world, but they are also more confused.

# 2 Sugar is not always sweet! 🍎

People LOVE sweet food. Even before humans started to refine sugar, we looked for food that tastes sweet. Breast milk is sweet which is why babies prefer sweet food. Grains, beans, vegetables and fruit all contain natural sugar which carries a variety of vitamins, minerals, enzymes and proteins that are good for us. When brown rice is cooked, chewed and digested, the sugar in it breaks down into separate glucose molecules, which enter the bloodstream and bring the body lots of good nutrients. Natural sugar is good for us and gives us long lasting energy.

## CAN YOU TELL THE DIFFERENCE BETWEEN EATING SUGAR IN FRUIT VERSUS SUGAR IN CANDY?

This is the difference between eating natural sugar and eating refined sugar. Refined, or processed, sugar is white. Processing separates the sugar from the fiber, vitamins and minerals, leaving it with hardly any nutrients. This makes it much more difficult for our bodies to digest the sugar properly. Refined sugar raises our blood sugar levels too quickly, giving us short bursts of energy. Without additional nutrients, our bodies can't sustain the energy burst and our blood sugar levels will crash, making us tired and cranky. When this happens, we crave more sugar and the cycle repeats itself. If this happens often, you can get sick. All serious diseases start as inflammation in the body and sugar feeds this inflammation. As if this wasn't enough, sugar also causes tooth decay and gum disease!

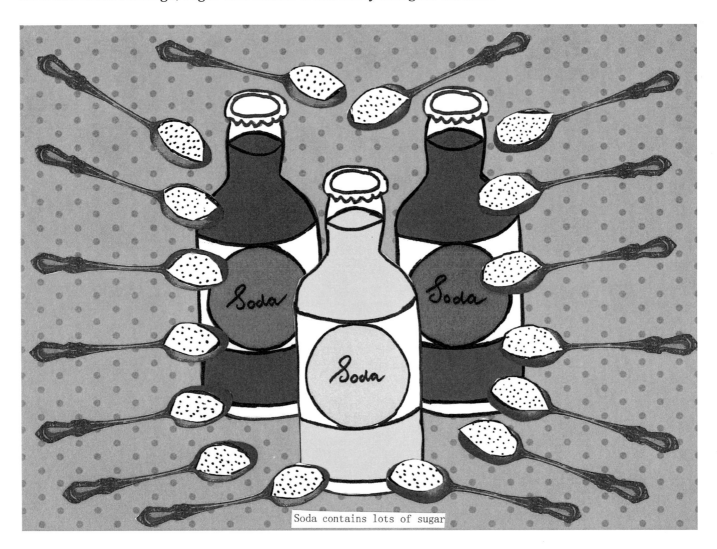

Soda contains lots of sugar

## HOW MUCH REFINED SUGAR DO YOU EAT IN A TYPICAL DAY?

The average American consumes more than 100 pounds of sugar each year! This is more than a quarter of a pound or 4 ounces per day which is equivalent to 26 teaspoons (4 grams each) or 52 sugar cubes (2 grams each)! The United States Department of Agriculture (USDA) recommends that we eat no more than 10 teaspoons or 20 cubes of sugar per day, but we eat almost three times as much as we should.

Eating sugar has always been part of our history, but we used to eat much less than we do now. In the 17th century, colonists ate only 4 pounds of sugar per year. They started eating more sugar after the first sugar refinery was built in NYC in 1689, and sugar no longer had to be imported from the Caribbean islands where it was grown. Eating four pounds of sugar a year would be the same as eating 1 sugar cube per day!

## REALLY?

You might think that you do not consume 52 sugar cubes (2 grams each) each day. Where is all this sugar coming from? You have to be a detective to find out where the sugar is hidden.

Most of the added sugar we eat today comes from sodas and other sweetened beverages. Manufacturers think that if they add more sugar to their products people will like them better and buy more! People who drink a lot of soda consume much more than the recommended amount of sugar per day.

# Soda

Let's examine a bottle of orange soda. The average size of a single serving is 20 ounces. On the label you might see an orange fruit and a green leaf. It says the drink is caffeine free, which is good. It also says the drink contains 100% natural flavors. It is easy to think that this soda is made of real oranges but this is just marketing to make you buy this product. If you turn the bottle and look at the "Nutrition Facts" label, it clearly says "CONTAINS NO JUICE" and when we look at the sugar content it says "74 grams per serving"!

Now do the math: two grams of sugar equals one sugar cube. If you divide 74 grams of sugar by 2, you get more than 37 cubes of sugar in this one serving alone! Look how easy it is to consume an enormous amount of sugar without even knowing it! And this is only one drink!

Let's see how much sugar you eat in a typical day, starting with breakfast. Many kids eat cereal for breakfast so we can use a fruity-o cereal as an example. The recommended serving size for cereal is one cup which is not very much. This small serving contains 12 grams of sugar which is 6 cubes of sugar. If you use low-fat milk on your cereal, you need to add another 13 grams per serving, or 6 1/2 cubes!

Many children like to have juice in the morning. One serving of orange juice contains 22 grams of sugar and most apple juice contains 24 grams. Let's add another 11 cubes of sugar to our total!

By mid-morning you're feeling a little hungry so you eat a snack. Let's assume you eat a healthy granola bar. The nutrition facts on the wrapper tell us that the average 'healthy' granola bar has 10 grams of sugar. This is close to 5 cubes of sugar to add to our total. We are now only mid-morning and we have already eaten more than 30 cubes of sugar which is more than the USDA thinks is good for us. We still have to eat lunch, an afternoon snack, dinner and dessert!

## WHAT ABOUT YOU?

> *Pick one day in the week to calculate how much sugar you consume.*
>
> 1. *List everything you swallowed and how much of it you ate.*
>
> 2. *Now add up all the sugar you consumed by calculating the equivalent number of sugar cubes for each item you ate or drank.*
>
> 3. *What do you see? What does this tell you about the food you are eating?*

Children are still growing and their bodies are getting bigger and stronger every day. Your body is growing because you are giving it the nutrients it needs from the good things you eat and drink. Your body uses these nutrients to make your arms and legs grow longer and stronger.

If your body is built from the nutrients you eat, would you prefer to grow from food with few nutrients, so-called 'empty' foods, or would you prefer your body to grow using food loaded with healthy vitamins and minerals? While you may not be able to choose everything you eat, you are able to make some very important nutritional decisions: drinking a glass of water or a soda, eating candy or a piece of fruit? Remember, all small changes you make, are big changes for your health now and in the future!

## DOES THIS MEAN CAN YOU NEVER EAT YOUR FAVORITE CHOCOLATE CHIP COOKIE AGAIN? OF COURSE YOU CAN!

Just remember the 90%-10% rule…. If you eat a healthy diet 90% of the time, you can have a sweet treat the rest of the time.

## TIP

If you want to eat something sweet, can you think of a better choice than a chocolate chip cookie? Fruit and vegetables like carrots and celery are also sweet. You can eat them instead.

Rather than drinking a soda, how about a glass of cold water? And if you like apple juice a lot, why don't you pour half a glass of apple juice and then add bubbly water and a fancy straw. It tastes just as good!

---

### RECIPE FOR THE BEST CHOCOLATE BANANA ICE CREAM

Before beginning any recipe, get an adult's permission to work in the kitchen. If your recipe uses knives, the stove, or other kitchen appliances, you must have some adult help! Although making food is fun, it's important to be safe!

You need:

- frozen bananas (it is easiest to peel the banana, cut it into slices and freeze it in a Ziploc bag until you need it)

- ¼ cup almond milk or coconut water

- 2 tablespoons of cacao powder

Blend ingredients in a high speed blender or food processor until they are as smooth as you like. Enjoy!

---

Let's review:

1. There is a difference between natural sugar and processed sugar.

2. It is easy to eat too much processed sugar.

3. Sugar is not always 'sweet' because it can be at the root of illnesses.

4. You can still have 'sweet' recipes without processed sugar!

# 3   We grow food, and food grows us

### *Food grows us!*

In the introduction chapter we talked about the phrase "you are what you eat". Our bodies are built from the nutrients we consume every day. Knowing this allows us to 'own', and take care of our health.

### Messages

Your body sends you messages all the time. Are you listening? Thirst is a message. What does it tell you? Hunger is a message? What does it tell you? Pain is also a message? What would happen if you didn't feel pain when you hurt yourself. Both hunger and thirst are the body's messages to the brain that more nutrients are needed for growth, maintenance, energy and repair! How does your body transform the foods you eat into the nutrients you need? In other words: how does food grow us?

> **The Swallowing Experiment**
>
> *Try this experiment to demonstrate how food travels through the esophagus to the stomach.*
>
> Take a sip of water and then bend over to touch your toes. Can you still swallow the water? Why?

# Digestion

This is the process of breaking food down into millions of tiny pieces. Digestion begins in your mouth, when you chew your food, and ends in the toilet, following a route about 30 feet, all inside your body! After you chew and swallow your food, it travels to the stomach by way of a tube called the **esophagus**. Food does not fall down the esophagus because of gravity; wave-like muscle-contractions carry the food to the stomach.

Imagine you are eating a sandwich for lunch. Take a bite, chew well and swallow. Once your food travels down your esophagus, it empties into your **stomach**, which is like a big bag. The stomach lining produces gastric juices which help to break down the food so your body can absorb it. If you have ever thrown up, you've tasted your gastric juices.

Yuk!

Most of the action of digestion occurs in the **small intestine**, which is a coiled-up organ that looks like a tube. The small intestine is about 20 feet long in kids, and a bit longer in adults. Enzymes found here help to break down your sandwich even more. The nutrients taken from the digested food in your stomach are pulled out through the walls of the small intestine and into the blood stream to be sent to different parts of your body.

All that's left of your lunch now is whatever your body can't use. This looks like a brown paste which collects in the *large intestine.* Here, water is added to the paste to make poop, which is excreted into the toilet. The digestion of your lunch is complete!

While food is broken down somewhat by chewing and grinding, most digestion happens because of body chemicals. These chemicals, known as enzymes, break down the food in the mouth, stomach and small intestine. Other chemicals include acid in the stomach, which helps to break down the food you just chewed and bile from the gall bladder which helps break down fat.

# Absorption

After food is digested into small particles, it must somehow move from the intestines to the rest of the body. That movement into the bloodstream is called absorption and happens mainly in the small intestine. The small intestine is made up of millions of fingerlike projections called villi. The villi are covered with a hair like brush that traps the nutrients. The nutrients are then passed through the villi into tiny blood vessels called capillaries which eventually empty into the body's major blood vessels.

# Circulation

How do nutrients find their way up to our noses and down to our toes? Every cell of the body requires a continuous supply of energy from nutrients we eat and oxygen from the air we breathe. Oxygen and nutrients are transported to the cells by arteries, while veins carry carbon dioxide and waste products out of the cells. This network of blood vessels, including the small, web like, connecting vessels we know as capillaries, make up the circulatory system. The circulatory system relies on a very important pump, the heart, to continually move blood through the body.

# Metabolism

Once nutrients finally make their way to the millions of tiny cells that make up the body, they are used to supply the building blocks for energy, healing, maintenance and growth. Each cell of the body is like a tiny factory, taking the raw materials of nutrition and producing energy or growth or replacement parts. At any given moment, the cells of an active child are busy supplying energy to run at recess, creating new cells to make bones and muscles bigger, sending sugar to the working brain, and producing skin cells to heal a scraped knee.

Fortunately, the body does all these things without you knowing it! The only thing you have to do is eat food that supplies the necessary raw materials. It really is true: You are what you eat!

So this is how your body, like a very well working factory, transforms the foods you eat into the nutrients for energy, growth, maintenance or repair. In other words: This is how food makes us grow!

Although this process works more or less the same for everybody (and *every* body), individual people react differently to foods.

# Bio-individuality

These differences have to do with where you were born (ancestry) and where you live (near the sea, in the mountains, where it's warm or where it's cold). It also has to do with your unique body. Some people cannot tolerate certain foods and get sick if they eat nuts, fish, gluten or dairy products. These are called food allergies or sensitivities. It is important to never judge people because of what they eat.

## DIETS

If you go into a bookstore you'll always see many books about new diets that promise you to lose weight or to make you healthier. But the reason diets don't work, at least not for everybody, for every body, is that every body has its own unique needs and its own unique reactions to diets and life styles.

So while most diets tell people what they should not eat, it is far more important to think about what healthy foods you can add to what you eat and drink on a daily basis. If you add more water, you'll crowd out sodas. If you add an apple a day, you'll crowd out one salty or sugary snack. Think of foods in a very positive way. Think about how certain foods can help your body grow in a healthy way. Add in healthier choices to crowd out unhealthier choices. This way your diet will be fun!

*Something to think about*

This chapter has as title "we grow food and food grows us". People have been growing food for thousands of years, but in the last century their methods of growing foods have changed enormously. This has influenced the food itself and we do not know yet to what extent this influences the way this food grows us. The next chapters will explain this in more detail.

Let's review:

1. Digestion is the process of breaking food down into millions of tiny pieces so the body can absorb the nutrients it needs to keep us healthy.

2. Bio-individuality means that every body is different and that our bodies react differently to all foods. Food we eat is a personal choice. It is never appropriate to judge people because of what they eat.

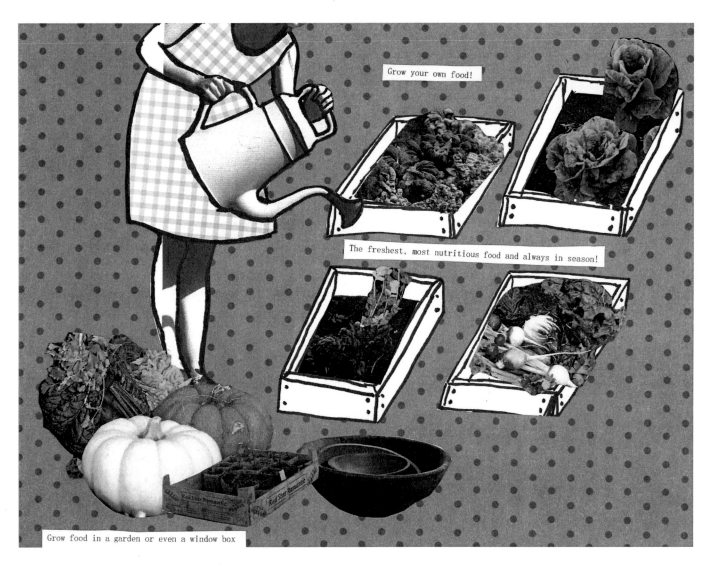

Grow your own food!

The freshest, most nutritious food and always in season!

Grow food in a garden or even a window box

# 4  About carbs, fats, proteins and eating your colors! 🍎

In the chapter about sugar we learned that the average American eats over 100 pounds of sugar a year. Do you know how many pounds of broccoli Americans eat? Not even 4 pounds! This is a real shame because vegetables are so good for us and they really do taste great. You just need to find your favorite way to eat them.... boiled, stir-fried, poached, steamed and even raw. However you eat them, vegetables are the best choice!

## Macro-nutrients and Micro-nutrients

When we talk of nutrition, we often speak about food groups. *Carbohydrates* form a food group. *Protein* forms another food group, and *Fats* form the last food group. Carbohydrates, proteins and fats are called macro-nutrients (macro means large), and you need large amounts of them in your diet. Micro nutrients, (micro means small), are vitamins and minerals. You need small amounts of micro nutrients in your diet. Vitamins and minerals make nutrients work together. Everything your body does is helped along by vitamins or minerals.

Eating some foods from each of the food groups is one way to get the nutrients you need to grow and be healthy.

**Carbohydrates** are the body's major source of energy. Foods like bread, corn, rice and potatoes are all carbohydrates.

**Protein** provides the building blocks you need to grow, maintain or replace body tissue. Some people think that eating animal protein such as beef, chicken and fish is the only way we can get the protein we need. Fortunately, you can also get protein from plants. The parts of a plant that can sprout and grow, such as seeds, dry beans and peas, nuts and grains, are also very good sources of protein!

**Fats** are another source of energy. Olive oil, nuts, avocados and fatty fish are all good sources of healthy fat. They help the body absorb certain vitamins and are good for your growing brain.

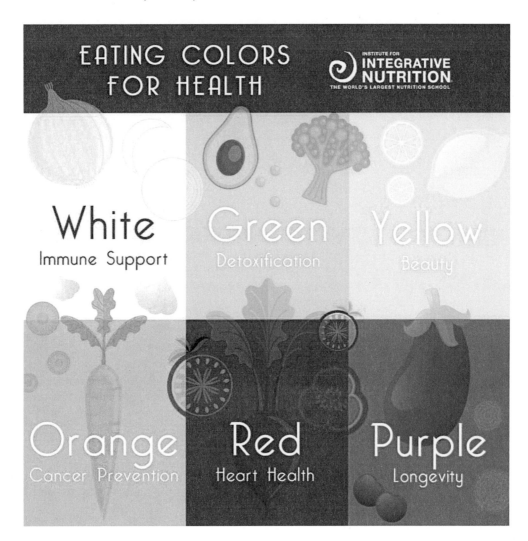

---

**WHAT ARE OXIDANTS, ANTI-OXIDANTS AND FREE RADICALS?**

OXIDANTS are very corrosive molecules that destroy everything they touch. Think of a rusty nail in an old piece of wood – the nail is being attacked by oxidants which cause it to rust and fall apart.

Every time you breathe, some of the oxygen you inhale breaks down into matter called FREE RADICALS. These free radicals are very corrosive and attack your body's cells. Our cells can't rust – they just die. When our cells die, we don't feel very well.

Thankfully, our body has a secret weapon to destroy these oxidants. They're called ANTI-OXIDANTS and we get many them from the food we eat. Some anti-oxidants work best in watery places like our blood, while others work best in fatty places like our cells. Eating different kinds of foods give us the different kinds of anti-oxidants we need to stay healthy. Fruits and vegetables are loaded with anti-oxidants.

---

A really fun way to get great nutrition is to eat food by color! Each color has a different health benefit, so sampling fruit and vegetables from each color makes a really healthy diet.

A colorful salad looks beautiful and is also great for you! If you eat as many different colors as you can, you'll make sure you get all the vitamins and minerals your body needs.

**Here are the most common food colors and the good things they give us. You can literally eat the rainbow!**

**White:** Foods that are white in color are wonderful for your immune system because they are anti-viral, anti-fungal, and anti-inflammatory, which helps the body fight infections. White fruits and vegetables raise good cholesterol and lower bad cholesterol to keep your heart healthy, and fight diseases that affect your immune system and cancer.

**Garlic, onions** and **cauliflower** are examples of white food. Can you think of any others?

**Green:** Dark leafy greens contain so many things your body needs: vitamins A and C, fiber and anti-oxidants that keep you from getting sick! Green food gets their color from chlorophyll (clor-o-fil) which helps to purify, or clean, your blood. They also contain lots of vitamin K which helps to build strong bones and to prevent your blood from clotting when it is not supposed to. Green fruit and vegetables are loaded with calcium and zinc which helps your body to grow strong and stay healthy.

Do you like any of these green foods? **Broccoli, kale, collards, asparagus, green beans, celery, lettuce** and **spinach?**

**Yellow:** Fruits and vegetables that are rich in Vitamin C are yellow in color. Eating them helps reduce swelling in your body, prevent allergies by boosting your immune system, and gives you healthy skin by helping your blood to circulate smoothly. Vitamin C also fights free radicals. Yellow foods taste great! They include **lemons** (think lemonade!!), **pineapples, yellow peppers**, and **grapefruit**.

**Orange:** These foods are orange because of a mineral called beta-carotene. Your body transforms the beta-carotene into Vitamin A and anti-oxidants to keep your eyes and skin healthy. These nutrients also help to prevent cancer, heart disease and infections.

The most famous orange fruit is the orange!! Other fruits and vegetables loaded with beta-carotene are: **cantaloupe, mangoes, sweet potatoes, carrots** and **squash**.

**Red:** The circulatory system and cells in your body get stronger when you eat red fruit and vegetables. This keeps your blood pressure at a safe level and helps your organs, like your heart, lungs and kidneys, working well. Red food also helps to improve your memory and acts like nature's sun screen by giving you protection from the sun's harmful ultra-violet rays.

Who doesn't love a bright **red tomato**, a slice of juicy **watermelon** or a bowl full of **cherries**? These are red foods. Other red foods include **beets** and **red peppers**, hot or sweet.

**Purple:** The anti-oxidant super heroes of the food world are the purple foods. They help you stay really healthy so you can live for a long time. They also raise your "good" cholesterol and keep your brain healthy and active.

Purple foods include **blueberries, blackberries, eggplant**, and **purple cabbage**.

*Let's review:*

1. *Fats, carbohydrates and proteins are macro-nutrients. Vitamins and minerals are micro-nutrients. We need both of these to stay healthy.*

2. *Carbohydrates and fats give us energy; protein provides the building blocks we need to grow. We can get all of these by eating fruits and vegetables.*

3. *Fruits and vegetables come in a rainbow of colors and we should eat some of each color every day.*

4. *Fruits and vegetables contain lots of important nutrients and vitamins. They also contain anti-oxidants which destroy the free radicals that can make us sick.*

5. *Because they are so powerful, fruits and vegetables should make up the biggest part of our diet.*

6. *Try eating your vegetables cooked different ways, or raw, to find out what tastes best to you.*

# 5   Whole food and processed food

What do you usually eat for breakfast? Eating a good breakfast is important because you'll need lots of energy for the day! Remember, you have not eaten anything substantial since dinner last night. What do you usually have for lunch, dinner and snacks? Do you know if you are eating whole food or processed food?

Whole foods look exactly the way they appear in nature. Processed foods are different from the way they look in nature, because they have been changed in a factory and are usually sold in a package.

Compare a raw potato and a bag of chips. The raw potato is unprocessed because that is how it is found in nature. When the potato is skinned, cut, fried, flavored, sealed in a bag and then shipped to a store for you to buy, we say that food has been processed.

## MANY PEOPLE BELIEVE THAT WHOLE FOODS ARE A BETTER CHOICE FOR YOUR HEALTH. DO YOU KNOW WHY?

Whole foods are great for you because they contain all the vitamins and minerals your body needs. Nothing has been taken away.

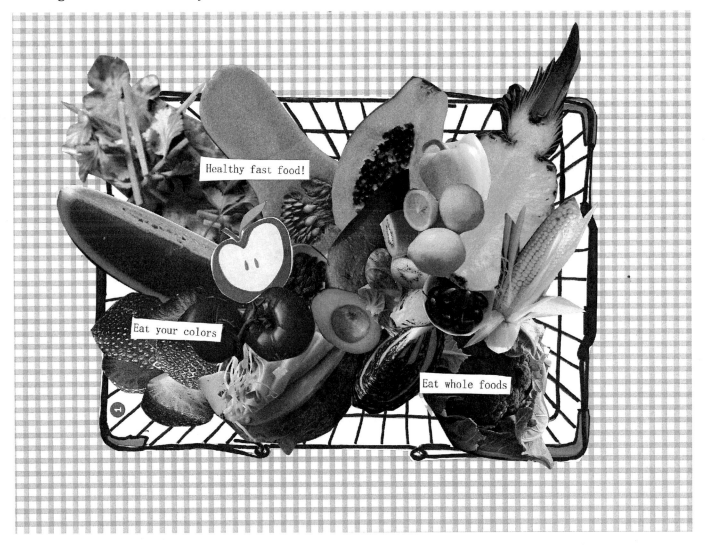

Let's look at some other examples of whole and processed food. Natural sugar is loaded with vitamins, enzymes and fiber. We can find natural sugar in fruits and vegetables.

Processed sugar, the white stuff, has been changed so much that none of these nutrients are left. Your body gets no benefits at all from eating it. The whole grains that go into whole grain bread also have lots of vitamins, minerals and fiber that your body loves and needs. White bread contains only processed grains which have been stripped of all these nutrients. It makes your tummy feel full, your brain sluggish and your body unhappy.

Your body needs whole food to stay healthy.

Do you remember the ingredient list for the bottle of orange soda or the nutrition snack bar? There are so many ingredients which most people do not recognize or understand. What is on the ingredient list of a banana? Just banana! What is on the ingredient list of broccoli? Just broccoli!

Processed foods not only have a lot of nutrients and fiber removed from them, there are a lot of strange ingredients added to them, too. Chemicals and food dyes are added to make your food look more attractive, or last longer. Those chemicals and food dyes make it possible for processed food to look and feel fresh for a long time, but they are NOT good for your health.

## HOW DO YOU THINK YOU CAN ADD MORE WHOLE FOODS TO YOUR DAILY DIET?

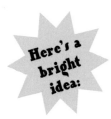
Here's a bright idea:

Add some fresh fruit to your breakfast cereal, eat an apple (skin and all) as a morning snack and enjoy some red peppers or carrots with a healthy dip for an afternoon snack. That wasn't hard!

# RED FLAG! High Fructose Corn Syrup (HFCS) and Trans Fats

If you see one of these two names on any package of processed food, you know for sure you should make a better, healthier choice.

High Fructose Corn Syrup, or HFCS, was completely unknown until about 30 years ago, but now every person in America consumes more than 65 pounds of it every year! Fructose is just sugar, but high fructose corn syrup is a very strong form of sugar that comes from corn. It is sweeter than regular sugar, it increases your appetite, and is very addictive. Because it makes you want to eat more than you need, it can lead to obesity, and diabetes. It can even cause an infection in your brain! You'll find HFCS in lots of processed and junk food, even your favorite ketchup!

Trans fats are found in processed foods, baked goods, most fried food and almost any product that comes from a factory. Trans fats damage cells and can also hurt your developing brain. They can raise the amount of cholesterol in your blood (bad!) and cause heart disease (even worse!).

Whole or processed food? Which one do you prefer?

*Let's review:*

1. *Unprocessed (whole) foods have not been changed from the way they are found in nature. Processed foods have been changed by skinning, chopping, cooking, adding extra ingredients or worse, dyes and chemicals to preserve them, and wrapping them in packages for sale.*

2. *Our bodies need unprocessed food to be healthy. Processed food has too many nutrients removed to be good for us.*

3. *If you see High Fructose Corn Syrup or trans fats listed as an ingredient in processed food you pick up at the supermarket, see if you can find a similar item without those.*

4. *Eating whole food, instead of processed food, means you avoid eating HFCS and trans fats.*

# 6  If we change food, food changes us 🍎

We know that the food we grow, grows us. It is also true that if we change or alter the basic structure of the food, it will change us. Let me explain.

For thousands of years people have been using very simple ways to grow food- a plow pulled by an animal to till the soil, a simple hoe to plant the seeds and lots of hard work to harvest the crops. In many parts of the world, farmers still grow food this way. When people grew more than they needed, they sold the rest so they could buy other things like clothes and supplies for their homes.

During the last 100 years, industrialization changed our lives in many ways. It also changed the way we grow food. Machines now do the work people and animals used to do. Today it is easier to grow and harvest much more food than one farmer can eat which has made more food available and cheaper to buy. Also, farmers now grow fewer varieties of fruits and vegetables, preferring to grow only one or two crops that earn the most money at market. This drains the soil of important nutrients so farmers have to add chemicals to make it possible to grow the same crops next season.

In the last century people made other changes to create bigger profits. Through genetic modification scientists change the structure of cells in plants to make them stronger, creating bigger harvests and bigger profits. These plants are called GENETICALLY MODIFIED ORGANISMS (GMOS). Furthermore, farmers now use chemical fertilizers to help crops grow in depleted soil, and chemical pesticides to make plants more resistant to disease or drought and to protect them from being eaten by bugs. While not all chemicals have been tested on humans, we know that high levels of pesticides can poison, or even kill, people. Pesticide residue that remains on unwashed fruit may cause diseases, and can affect a developing child's brain.

*If we are what we eat, we should expect that if we change the food we eat, that food will change us, too.*

One way to avoid eating these chemicals is to buy 'organic' food when we shop for groceries.

## WHAT DOES IT MEAN TO BE "ORGANIC"?

'Organic' is a strange label because all food is organic. It just means it is made from living things. When you go shopping today, you might see vegetables in one aisle of the produce section labeled 'conventionally grown', and in another aisle, 'organic'. 'Conventionally grown' food is another confusing term. Maybe 'grown using chemicals' would be a better way to describe them.

Is there really a difference between organic and conventionally grown fruit and vegetables? Organic produce looks the same as fruit and vegetables produced through conventional farming, but there are differences.

Organic farmers do not use pesticides to help their crops grow or to protect them from disease. Instead they use compost and animal manure to fertilize the soil and they add complementary crops to keep the plants safe from bugs and disease. Organic farming is friendly to our planet and the wonderful diversity of living things on it.

When you buy organic food, you support something called **sustainable farming**. This type of farming is the way people used to farm when your grandparents were children. If a farmer grows grains one year, the next year he will grow a different crop, and then the next year something different again and then the fourth year he may let the soil rest so it can restore its minerals and nutrients.

With organic foods it is most important to consider what is NOT in it. The real difference between conventional farming and organic farming is that no unhealthy sprays or pesticides are used in the production of organic food. When organic food is cooked and sold in supermarkets, no preservatives are added to artificially prolong its freshness. The longer food stays on the shelves in the supermarket or in your kitchen cupboard, the less nutritious it becomes.

When buying food, you have the choice to pick a good, better or best option. For example, if you have the choice between a carrot candy and a real carrot, a good choice would be the real carrot. An even better choice would be an organic carrot, and the best choice is to pick a fresh, organic carrot that has been grown on a farm near you.

Fresh foods are best because they contain the most nutrients. A carrot that has been in your fridge for a couple of weeks loses many of its nutrients. Food that is produced on farms across the country or on farms in another country must travel many miles to get to your plate. During the transport from the farm to your supermarket, much of the nutritional value of the food is lost so food grown nearby is much better for you.

Remember, the best of the best is ORGANIC, fresh, in season and locally grown! It is not as difficult as it sounds, but organic food can be more expensive. For this reason sometimes you have to choose which foods to buy organic and which foods not to buy organic. But is organic food always healthy? In its raw form, it is the healthiest food to eat. But if the organic ingredients have been processed into something else, like a cookie, is it still healthy for us? A cookie contains lots of sugar and we know how unhealthy too much sugar can be. So, organic cookies are better than non-organic ones, but unprocessed organic food is best.

Let's review:

1. Modern, or conventional farming uses chemicals to produce more food. These farms often grow only one or two crops to increase the amount of money they make.

2. Genetically modified plants are resistant to disease and produce high yields, but may not be healthy for us to eat.

3. Organic farming uses compost and manure to increase yields and rotates crops to keep the soil healthy. Organic farmers never use chemicals on their plants.

4. Organic food can be more expensive than conventionally grown fruit and vegetables, so it's important to remember the good, better and best options: fresh fruit and vegetables are good, organic ones are better, and locally grown organic crops are best.

5. If organic crops are processed into sweet treats, they are no longer considered healthy.

# 7   How to know? Get the know how!

## Food marketing and nutrition facts

If you want to make healthier food choices, you have to understand food labels. Many packaged foods come with deceiving messages. Do you remember the misinformation we found on the bottle of orange soda and box of breakfast cereal in Chapter 1? "Fruit" candy, that contains no actual fruit, is another example of marketing misinformation. These marketing schemes are created by manufacturers to get you to buy their products. The information they present may or may not be true and it is up to us to figure it out.

To make healthy choices, you need nutrition know-how!

## *Food marketing*

Marketing is used when food companies want to sell their products, but you have to be aware that marketing uses language that might be misleading, or even untrue. The front of a box or a product label is where the company markets the product to us, the consumer. It's like a commercial on television, except it doesn't move. To get the attention of children, the box might show you cartoon figures you like. If it wants to show you that it is good for your health, it might show images of fruit and vegetables, or people doing sports. However, printing a picture of an orange on the label does not necessarily mean that the contents of the bottle contains real orange juice. Remember the image of the orange on the orange soda label? We might think that orange soda contains real orange juice but the bottle's nutrition facts state clearly that the drink "contains no juice". Only if we read these nutrition facts we will know the true facts about nutrition!

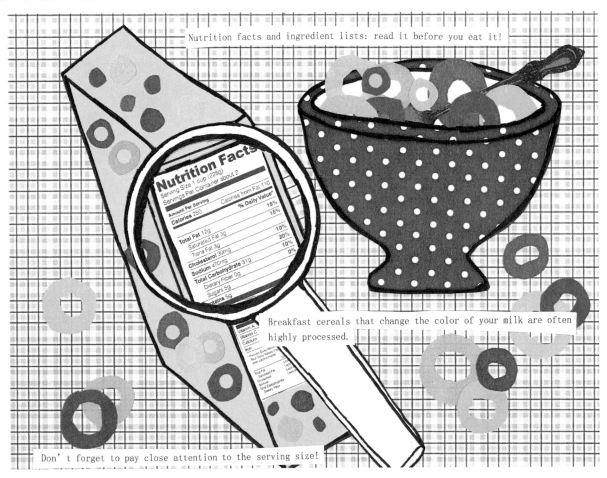

Nutrition facts and ingredient lists: read it before you eat it!

Breakfast cereals that change the color of your milk are often highly processed.

Don't forget to pay close attention to the serving size!

## *Nutrition facts tell you the facts about nutrition*

The Nutrition Facts label, found on all packaged food, contains valuable information for making healthy food choices at the grocery store. Here are a few things you should look for.

Check the **serving size** of your favorite packaged snack like a box of cookies, a bowl of cereal or some canned fruit. The serving size tells you how much is in a serving and how many servings there are in that container.

Measure one serving size of your favorite snack. This might include counting the number of cookies in one serving or pouring a serving of cereal into a measuring cup. You may find that what the food manufacturer thinks is a reasonable serving is much less than you actually eat.

The **number of calories** listed on the label measures the amount of energy you get from eating a serving of that food.

The **amount per serving** tells you how many calories there are in each serving and how many of those calories come from fat. If you eat two servings, you'll be eating twice the number of calories listed on the box. However, food low in calories does not necessarily mean that it is healthy. The saying "calories are calories" is not true. Compare 200 calories that come from cookies with 200 calories that come from broccoli. Are these calories equally healthy?

Now look at what is listed under **fat, cholesterol, sodium (salt) and sugar** on the label. These are the not-so-healthy ingredients in packaged food. We should eat these only in small amounts because they can cause weight gain and other health problems.

**Nutrition Facts**

Serving Size 1 cup (228g)
Servings Per Container about 2

**Amount Per Serving**

| Calories 250 | Calories from Fat 110 |
|---|---|

**% Daily Value***

| | |
|---|---|
| **Total Fat** 12g | 18% |
| Saturated Fat 3g | 15% |
| *Trans* Fat 3g | |
| **Cholesterol** 30mg | 10% |
| **Sodium** 470mg | 20% |
| **Total Carbohydrate** 31g | 10% |
| Dietary Fiber 0g | 0% |
| Sugars 5g | |
| **Proteins** 5g | |

| | |
|---|---|
| Vitamin A | 4% |
| Vitamin C | 2% |
| Calcium | 20% |
| Iron | 4% |

* Percent Daily Values are based on a 2,000 calorie diet. Your Daily Values may be higher or lower depending on your calorie needs:

| | Calories: | 2,000 | 2,500 |
|---|---|---|---|
| Total Fat | Less than | 65g | 80g |
| Saturated Fat | Less than | 20g | 25g |
| Cholesterol | Less than | 300mg | 300mg |
| Sodium | Less than | 2,400mg | 2,400mg |
| Total Carbohydrate | | 300g | 375g |
| Dietary Fiber | | 25g | 30g |

Locate **fiber, vitamins and minerals**, the "good" nutrients. These nutrients need to be eaten in larger amounts because they make the body stronger and can help you grow.

The last section on the Nutrition Facts label lists the **Percentages Daily Value** of a number of vitamins and minerals such as Vitamin A, Calcium and Iron. These numbers help determine if the food in the package has a high or low amount of a specific nutrient. If the daily value of the vitamin or mineral is less than 5%, the food is low in that nutrient; if it is greater than 20%, it contains lots of it.

If you look at a box of dry pasta, one serving may contain 0% of your daily requirement of calcium, but 25% of your daily requirement of the vitamin folate. It would be a good idea to add some leafy green vegetables or fish to your pasta because they contain lots of calcium. Eating a serving of pasta also means that you don't need to drink more orange juice today. Orange juice contains lots of folate, and your pasta lunch has just given you all the folate you need today.

## Ingredient lists

Below the Nutrition Facts label you will find a list of ingredients. This list tells you all the ingredients used to make the food inside the package. The main ingredient is listed first. If sugar is listed as one of the first three ingredients you'll know that the food contains a lot of sugar.

*Let's review:*

1. *Food manufacturers can make us think that their product is healthy to eat by putting pictures of fresh fruit and vegetables or healthy people on their packaging. We can only know if the product is healthy for us by reading the nutrition facts on the package.*

2. *Not all calories are equal. 200 calories from fruit or vegetables is better for you than 200 calories from cookies.*

3. *Eat only small amounts of sugar, fat, sodium and cholesterol and eat more food high in fiber, minerals and vitamins.*

4. *The more ingredients listed on the label, the more processed the food. Eat only food made with ingredients you can recognize and pronounce!*

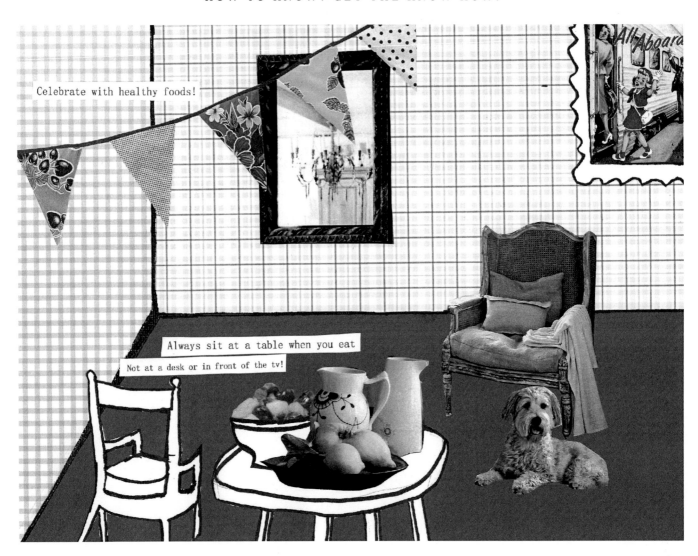

Celebrate with healthy foods!

Always sit at a table when you eat

Not at a desk or in front of the tv!

# 8  Nutrition and nourishment 🍎

*"Health is a state of complete physical, mental and social well-being and not merely the absence of disease or infirmity."* That's how the World Health Organization in Geneva, Switzerland describes good health. This is often cited as the official definition of good health since it was created in 1948!

We know that health is a vehicle and not a destination! Excellent health is about more than just not feeling sick. Good health allows us to be active, happy and have more fun.

## *Food Pyramids*

Food pyramids are nutritional diagrams in the shape of a pyramid. They are designed to show us how to make better food choices. The pyramid breaks food categories into a spectrum so you can have lots of variety in your diet. It is recommended that we eat more food from the wider sections, like grains, fruits and vegetables, and less food from the smaller sections like fats and sweets. But is nutrition the only way to keep us healthy?

Let's compare two different food pyramids. One is made by the USDA and the other is made by the Institute for Integrative Nutrition (IIN).

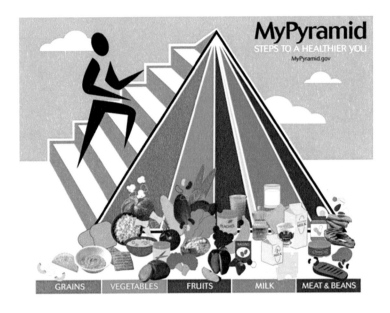

The USDA food pyramid (left) shows the different food groups and a figure running up the stairs. He represents exercise.

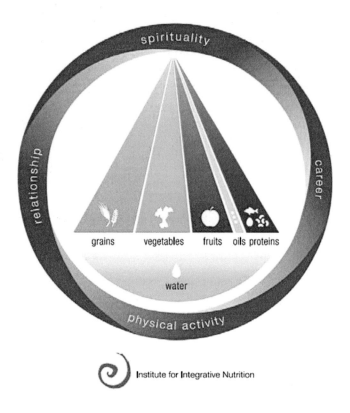

Institute for Integrative Nutrition

The IIN food pyramid (right) is a little different. It shows us that in addition to good nutrition, there are more things that nourish us and make us healthy. We need water to drink. Water is nature's best drink for us and we need plenty of it each day. To feel well mentally and socially we also need good relationships, like those we have with our family and friends. We need to believe that we make a difference in the world; that we matter. We also benefit greatly from spirituality. Spirituality is when we connect with something greater than ourselves. Some people find this connection in their church while others find it in other places. Love, success and spirituality are also forms of nutrition, a way to feed ourselves at a much deeper level than food alone.

This circle shows the major areas of your life. Let's rate how well you feel about things today.

Look at each section of the circle and identify each of the areas that are part of your life.

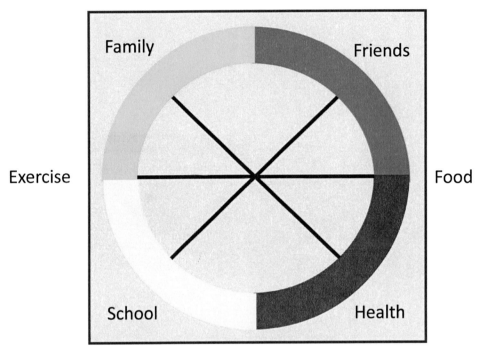

*The IIN Health Life Circle*

Place a dot on the line in each colored section to show how you feel about that part of your life. The closer to the outside of the circle, the better you feel right now. If you're not feeling so happy about this part of your life today, place the dot closer to the inside of the circle.

After you make six marks, one in each section, connect the dots. If your circle is round, you probably have a balanced, healthy life. If your circle is not so round, this shows you where you need to put some extra effort to create more balance and joy in your life.

The IIN Health Life circle is a wonderful exercise to see how the different areas of your life affect you. You can see if the different components are well-balanced, and you will have a clear visual of any imbalances. This can be a starting point for determining where you may want to spend more time and energy to create balance and joy in your life!

Use this exercise multiple times and write the dates you complete it on the back. If you use different colors for the different dates you complete this exercise, you will be able to clearly see any changes. To work on positive changes, think of simple ways you can improve how the different components work for you. For example, set simple, small and easily attainable goals. If you want to exercise more, try to walk to school one time a week or play outside more often. If you want to improve your friendships, you might set a goal to ask a friend for a play date or simply give someone a well-meant compliment. Positive change comes in many ways and in small steps!

Making the healthiest choices in the food we eat and drink are important elements in keeping us feeling great! Other factors which are just as important in keeping us healthy are finding happiness and purpose in our lives. We can accomplish this by strengthening our relationships and building successes.

*Let's Review:*

1. *Excellent health is about more than just not feeling sick. Good health allows us to be active, happy and have more fun.*

2. *Food pyramids are designed to show us how to make better food choices. It is recommended that we eat more food from the wider sections, like grains, fruits and vegetables, and less food from the smaller sections that include oils and sugar.*

3. *Good nutrition is not the only thing we need to keep us healthy. We also need exercise, love, success and spirituality.*

4. *The IIN Health Life circle is a good exercise to see how the different areas of your life affect you. This can be a starting point for determining where you may wish to spend more time and energy to create balance and joy in your life!*

# 9   Toxins in, on and around us 🍎

Just as we care about what we put INTO our bodies, we must be just as aware of the things we put ON our bodies, and the things that are AROUND our bodies.

These ingredients can also be harmful to our health. They are called 'toxins'.

---

**Toxins in Shampoo and Body Lotion**

*Parabens* and *Phthalates* are both toxins that are often found in shampoo and other cosmetics. They help to make the scent of the shampoo or lotion last longer or to keep the texture of a cosmetic soft, like lipstick. They are absorbed by our skin and find their way into our blood-stream. They can affect our growth and development and even make us very sick.

It is always better to buy shampoo that clearly states on the label **"Contains NO parabens and phthalates"**. This way, you avoid using products that you know contain toxins that are not good for you.

---

Toxins *IN* us are toxins that we ingest through food and water.

Toxins *ON* us are toxins that we absorb through our skin.

Toxins *AROUND* us are toxins that we inhale from our environment.

We feel our best when we eat well, exercise, are happy, and live in a healthy environment. However, toxins hide in so many places that we need to know where to find them so we can better protect ourselves.

**Toxins IN us.** We know that buying organic crops is better than buying fruit and vegetables that have been sprayed with toxic chemicals to make them grow faster. If you can't always buy organic, it is important to remember to always wash these toxins off before eating any fresh produce. This reduces the amount of toxins you ingest when you eat and drink non-organic food.

**Toxins ON us.** Our heart, lungs and stomach are all organs inside our bodies. This may surprise you, but skin is also an organ and it is your body's biggest one!

After you get out of bed in the morning, do you take a shower and wash your hair? Do you use toothpaste when you brush your teeth? Do you ever put lotion or sunscreen on your skin? Does your mom use a little make-up or ever spray on some perfume?

All of these body care products get absorbed through our skin and find their way into our bloodstream. Sometimes manufacturers put ingredients in their products to make them look pretty (like dyes to change their color), smell good by adding chemicals to mimic nice aromas, and even more chemicals to keep the products fresh longer.

These additional ingredients are also **toxins**.

How do you know if your body lotion contains toxins? Read the ingredient labels, just like you did with your food and drink choices. Remember, the fewer the ingredients, the better. If it contains too many ingredients that you cannot pronounce, put it back on the shelf and try something else.

## *Disinfecting*

Have you ever used an antiseptic gel to disinfect your hands? These gels kill almost all the bacteria that are found on the skin. That may sound like a good thing, but killing ALL the bacteria means you are also killing the good bacteria that live there. Good bacteria are necessary to keep your immune system strong so you can fight off infections. If you kill the good bacteria, along with the bad ones, you are at risk of becoming sick.

Read the ingredients listed on the label of the disinfectant bottle. Can you pronounce all the words? If not, perhaps you should look for another way to clean your hands. How about washing your hands with water?

## Toxins *AROUND* you

You spent a lot of time indoors at school and at home in rooms that are cleaned regularly. Have you ever read the ingredient labels on the cleaning supplies you use at home? Many actually contain warnings about the dangers of getting these products on our skin or in our eyes and warn us to be careful handling these products by using words like: CAUTION, WARNING and DANGER! We cannot take for granted that these products are safe to use.

Most commercial cleaning products are actually very bad for us. Their labels say they kill 99% of all germs, but remember, that includes both good and bad bacteria. Killing good bacteria leaves us unable to fight infections that we might contract and that's not good for our health. These commercial products are also more expensive.  Now the good news is that it is very easy to clean just about everything in your house with just two or three ingredients that are readily available in most kitchen cupboards. Instead of buying expensive and toxic cleaning products, you can make safe, effective and inexpensive cleaning supplies yourself! Just mix same amounts of water and white vinegar with an optional drop of lemon or an essential oil to make your own multipurpose cleaner.

The topic of toxins is broad and complex, but all you really need to remember is the following:

- To prevent toxins IN you, **choose organic** food and read the labels and nutrition facts of any processed food you buy.

- To prevent toxins ON you, read the ingredient list of any products you use on your skin such as shampoos and lotions and **choose the ones that say "Contains NO parabens and phthalates".**

- To reduce the amount of toxins AROUND you, read the ingredients in your cleaning supplies and choose the ones with the fewest chemicals. Better still, **make your own.**

Remember every little improvement you make, helps. You won't be able to change everything at once, so focus only on the things you <u>can</u> change. Be educated and informed, so you worry less about the things you can't change!

*Let's Review:*

1. *Toxins IN you are toxins that you ingest through food and water.*

2. *Toxins ON you are toxins that you absorb through your skin.*

3. *Toxins AROUND you are toxins that you inhale from your environment.*

4. *The fewer toxins you eat or touch, the healthier you will be.*

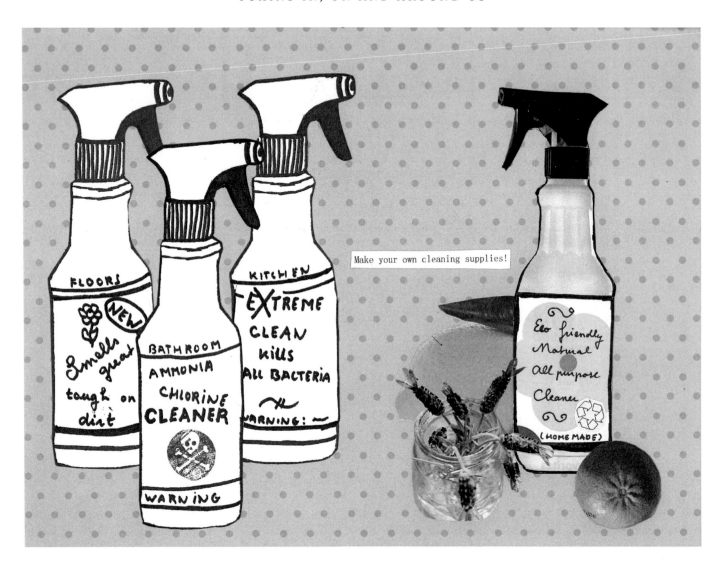

Make your own cleaning supplies!

# 10　Let's go shopping! 🍎

A trip to the grocery store will help you understand how difficult it can be to make healthy choices. There is so much food available in most supermarkets. Some of it is good, but a lot of it is bad for us. Choosing the best food for your budget can be really tough. Some guidelines can make your supermarket visits a bit easier.

## Organic markets

A number of markets offer organic food: MOM, Whole Foods and Trader Joe's are examples.

Let's look at MOM's market. MOM stands for My Organic Market. They sell food that is both organic and sustainable, and when possible, grown locally. The store tries to educate its customers to help them make better, healthier choices. MOM is really ahead of the game. Even their receipts are free of toxins.

# Farmers markets

Farmers markets are held in your area every day of the week. You can Google "*local farmers markets*" to find the one that is closest to your house. Farmers markets sell fresh, local produce as well as freshly baked bread and pastries. Usually the person selling the produce works on the farm where it was grown. Supporting our local farmers is really important if we want these small farms to survive. Remember though, not all produce sold at farmers markets is organic. Just make sure to ask the farmers if they used pesticides, and thoroughly wash whatever you buy before you eat it!

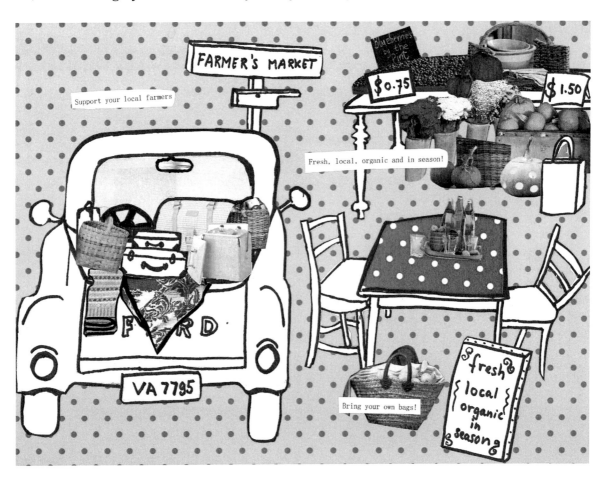

# Other grocery stores

If you shop at other grocery stores, here are some guidelines to keep in mind:

- **Shop the outer walls of the supermarket and stay out of the middle aisles.**

Most supermarkets display fresh food like fruit and vegetables, meat, dairy and fish along the outer walls of the store. Processed food is found in the center aisles.

- **Buy real food**

Real food is whole food. The ingredients in real food are as close to their natural state as possible. Real food generally contains no more than 5 ingredients. The more ingredients there are in packaged food, the more processed it is.

- **Avoid foods that say 'lite/light' or 'low-fat'**

These foods are not healthier for you. Whatever calories they give up in fats, they more than make up for in sugar.

- **Choose whole grains instead of refined grains or multi grains**

White bread is not healthy because all the nutritional parts of the wheat have been removed. That is why it is white and not wheat colored. Multigrain breads do not necessarily contain whole grains.

- **Stick to ingredients you can pronounce**

If you cannot pronounce the ingredient, don't eat it.

- **Don't buy imitation food**

Artificial sweeteners and imitation cheese such as Velveeta are examples. They require too much processing to be good for us.

- **Look at the labels and stickers on the food you buy**

If something is organic it should have a USDA certified organic label. It looks like this:

*Organic food* is produced without synthetic pesticides and has not been genetically modified. Organic meat and poultry are raised without hormones and antibiotics. These animals have been humanely reared and slaughtered.

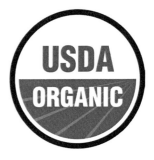

Many fruits and vegetables bought in food markets are marked with numbered stickers. If a product is organic, the number on this sticker will begin with 9.

## COOL : Country Of Origin Label

Fresh fruit, vegetables and meat often have a label indicating where the food was grown. Looking for this information allows you to see how many miles your food travelled to get to your plate. Food begins to lose some of its nutritional value as soon as it is picked. The longer the food is in a truck on the way to your supermarket, the less nutritious it becomes. Buying local products ensures that you get the most nutritious food you can. 'Local' means that it was grown or reared within a 100 mile radius from where you live.

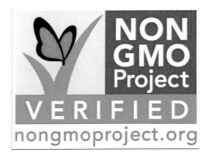

*GMO means Genetically Modified Organism*. This means that the plants have not developed naturally, but have been created in a laboratory to make them look perfect and travel long distances without rotting. When buying fresh fruit and vegetables, look for this label to ensure it is not genetically modified:

- **Bring your Dirty Dozen/ Clean Fifteen list**

The Dirty Dozen list identifies 12 fruits and vegetables grown using the greatest amount of chemical fertilizer and pesticides. These items are not organic. If you do buy any, you must wash them carefully before you eat them to remove any harmful chemicals.

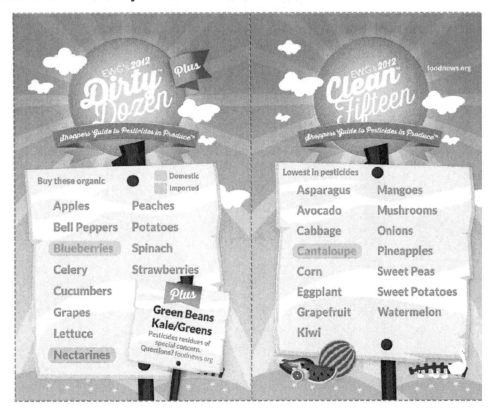

The Clean Fifteen list identifies 15 fruits and vegetables grown using limited amounts of chemical fertilizer and pesticides. Many of these items naturally have a protective skin or covering which is removed before the food is eaten, such as corn on the cob, onions or watermelon. This list is updated every year so check www. ewg.gov to get the latest version of the Dirty Dozen/ Clean Fifteen list from the *Environmental Working Group* in Washington, *D.C.*

*Let's Review:*

1. *There are many different places to buy fresh food, from local farmers markets to big supermarkets.*

2. *When possible buy real food grown locally.*

3. *When shopping in a supermarket, choose food found along the outer walls of the store. This is where you find fresh food. Stay away from the inside aisles which contain processed food.*

4. *Buy food made with ingredients you can pronounce.*

5. *Read the labels and stickers on the food you buy. They give you lots of important information about the food's level of nutrition.*

6. *Carry an updated copy of the Dirty Dozen/Clean Fifteen list to help you make informed food choices.*

7. *Food shopping is not always easy. Just remember, practice makes perfect.*

# 11   Helping to cook, cooking to help!

Cooking food is lots of fun. Do you ever help your parents prepare meals? Do you have a special dish that you know how to prepare yourself? Cooking our own food is not only good for our health, it also helps our environment. That is what we mean by "cooking to help".

## COOKING TO HELP.

We know that good nutrition is an important part of good health and part of good nutrition is to cut back on the amount of processed food we eat. As a nation, we are losing our ability to cook good, simple food at home, food that is cooked from "scratch", not from a box or frozen package.

We also know that if we are informed customers and consumers, we know how to buy real food- food that is fresh, local, in season, and if possible, organic. Preparing our own fresh food would send a message to food manufacturers that we want to eat healthy food, not processed food loaded with sugar, chemicals and preservatives. Our environment would be better for it, and so would we.

## HELPING TO COOK AND BEING SAFE IN THE KITCHEN.

Although making food is fun, it's important to know how to cook safely. This means knowing how to keep our workspace clean, how to use the appliances and tools safely, and when to ask for the help of an adult.

First, before beginning any cooking adventure, get an adult's permission to work in the kitchen and to use the appliances there. If your recipe uses knives, the stove, or other kitchen appliances that could be dangerous, you must have some adult help. When you have your helper there, you can avoid surprises, stay safe, and have fun while you cook.

## Find an Apron

Wearing an apron will keep your clothes clean. If you don't have an apron, an old shirt will do, but don't wear anything that's too big and loose. Baggy clothes can catch fire or get caught in kitchen tools like mixer beaters or the handle on a pot of boiling water.

## Germs

To keep germs from contaminating your food, it is important to keep the kitchen and your hands clean. Germs can contaminate your food which can make you sick. Always wash your hands with soap and water immediately before you begin cooking. Don't forget to clean under your fingernails too. This is especially important for recipes that involve touching the food directly, like kneading dough and mixing ingredients with your hands or handling animal flesh such as fish or chicken. You can also fight germs by keeping your working surfaces clean and dry. When you're finished cooking, always wash the countertops and any cutting boards you used with warm water before putting them away.

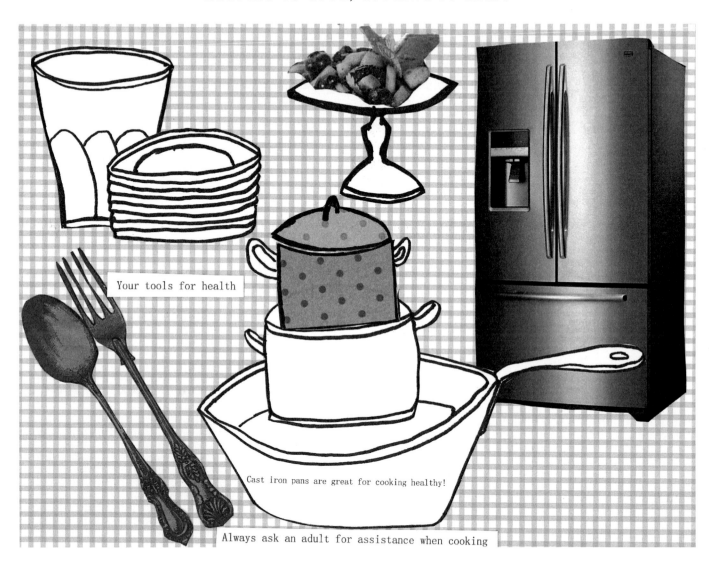

Your tools for health

Cast iron pans are great for cooking healthy!

Always ask an adult for assistance when cooking

## Stay safe

The best way to stay safe in the kitchen is to give the job your full attention. A kitchen is not a place to play. Too many accidents happen when people do not focus on the job at hand. After you wash your hands, dry them thoroughly. Wet hands are slippery and slippery hands cause accidents. If you have long hair, tie it back. This enables you to see clearly as you work and prevents your hair from catching on fire, or falling into the food you're cooking! Roll up your sleeves to keep them out of the ingredients and away from hot surfaces.

Kitchens have many hot surfaces that can easily burn you if you are not careful. Here are a few to remember. Sometimes it is not apparent that a stove burner, which has been turned off, is still hot to touch. Take note of the appliance's warning lights and keep your hands clear of the hot surfaces. A hot oven gives a burst of very hot air when you open the oven door. Keep your hands and face clear of the oven when opening it. Hot steam can also come from boiling liquid in cooking pots. Always open the lid away from your face to avoid getting burned by the steam. Remember that the handles on cooking pots can also be hot. Keep pot handles facing in and over counter and stove tops, and use a pot holder to protect your hand when moving them.

Stove tops have different sized burners to save electricity and prevent accidental burning. Remember to use a small burner for a small pot and a large burner for a large pot. Heating a small pot on a large burner wastes electricity and can burn you by exposing the hot burner as well as overheating the pot handle.

Blenders and food processors have very sharp moving parts. Always keep your fingers away from these blades when using these appliances. Kitchen knives are very sharp. Always point a knife blade away from yourself when handling it and keep your fingers away from the blade when you're cutting. When you are finished using the knife, clean it and put it away. A sharp knife in a sink of soapy water will surely cut the dishwasher's hand.

On a side note: microwave ovens are not a healthy choice preparing or thawing food, since the electromagnetic waves diminish the nutrients in your food. If you really have to use a microwave oven, never cover the food with foil or metal. This causes the microwaves to spark which can start a fire.

Clean up as you go. A messy kitchen increases your chances of spills and accidents. If you spill something on the floor, clean it up immediately so nobody slips and falls.

---

**LET'S GET COOKING!**

Recipe for healthy pancakes (gluten-free, vegan)

Ingredients:

- One banana

- One cup of gluten-free rolled oats

- One cup of almond milk

- One tablespoon of olive oil or coconut oil

Mix the first three ingredients in a blender. Put the oil in the pan and prepare as you would prepare pancake batter.

---

Let's Review:

1. Cooking our own food is the best way to eat real food. Cooking for ourselves helps us, and the plant, stay healthy.

2. Cooking is not difficult and is really fun!

3. The kitchen can be a dangerous place so it is important to be focused when cooking and be careful with hot appliances and sharp tools.

4. Keeping the kitchen and your tools clean is the best way to keep our food and kitchen germ free.

# 12   An appetite for health and happiness!

This book provides you with the skills and tools to make better and more educated choices for your health. You now know **you** can do a lot to support your health by knowing the facts about your nutrition. As 'health is wealth', that's great news!

Your parents may have told you not to play with your food on your plate, but you can still play with your food the following way: suppose all the kids in your class are having colds and are sniffing all day. What color food should you eat extra to help you protect your health? If pancakes are your favorite for breakfast, you now know a recipe for a healthier version of pancakes! The same goes for 'ice cream'! Suppose you have practiced soccer really hard because you want to help your team win the soccer game: what foods support your body? Now you know why the popular 'sports drink' depicting active people and many promises about fruits on the label is not really a good idea when you instead read the nutrition facts, learning that this 'sports drink' contains 'no real fruit juice' and contains 74(!) grams of sugar per serving. You know that this kind of processed sugar only makes your energy levels crash. Now you know that instead you need a real piece of fruit with natural, sustainable sugar and some water, you are ready to take on the game!

Long before you were born Hippocrates (born himself 460 BC) said : "Let food be thy medicine and medicine be thy food". As you are just starting your lives, my sincere wish for you is that you develop an appetite for health and happiness!

37932289R00049

Made in the USA
San Bernardino, CA
27 August 2016